Copyright © 2020

R.D.N

All rights reserved. No part of this publication may be reproduced, distributed, or transmitted in any form or by any means, including photocopying, recording, or other electronic or mechanical methods, without the prior written permission of the publisher, except in the case of brief quotations embodied in critical reviews and certain other non-commercial uses permitted by copyright law

Table of Contents

Introduction to Hypothyroidism diet 7

- Iodine 10
- Selenium 11
- Zinc 13
- Tips for weight loss with hypothyroidism 20

Hypothyroidism and Weight Loss Diet 23

- Consult with your Personal Doctor or Dietitian first: 25
- Thyroid hormone should be consumed fasting: 25
- Goitrogens, Soy and Legumes: 26
- Choose water as your drink: 26

Flexibility is key: 27

Limit or eliminate junk foods and highly processed products: 27

Day 1: Monday 28

Day 2: Tuesday 30

Day 3: Wednesday 31

Day 4: Thursday 31

Day 5: Friday 32

Day 6: Saturday 33

Day 7: Sunday 34

Hypothyroidism meal plan: 7 days 35

Monday 36

Tuesday 36

Wednesday 37

Thursday 37

Friday 38

Saturday 38

Sunday 39

Hypothyroidism Treatment | Natural Alternatives to Try 39

How to Lower Your Risk of Hypothyroidism 51

1. Manage Stress 51

2. Minimize Sugar Consumption 53

3. Avoid Gluten in Your Hypothyroidism Diet . 54

4. Watch Out for Perchlorates 55

5. Quit Smoking 55

6. Perform a Thyroid Neck Check 56

7. See Your Physician Regularly 57

Banana Turmeric Peanut Butter 60

Turmeric Tea Recipe For A Healthy Thyroid 62

Strawberry-Almond-Coconut Smoothie 67

Cocoa Bliss Smoothie 68

Watercress Green Juice 69

Rosemary Roasted Potatoes and Tomatoes 70

Baked Risotto Primavera 73

Southwestern Steak and Peppers 77

Sizzled Citrus Shrimp 81

Ginger-Chicken Noodle Soup 85

Green Beans With Bacon and Hazelnuts 87

Smoky Stuffed Peppers 90

Introduction to Hypothyroidism diet

Hypothyroidism occurs when the body does not produce enough thyroid hormones. Often, doctors treat hypothyroidism with medicine that replaces the thyroid hormones.

The thyroid is a small, butterfly-shaped gland in the throat. Having hypothyroidism, or an underactive thyroid, can slow down metabolism, cause weight gain, and cause fatigue.

A person's diet can have a significant impact on the symptoms of hypothyroidism. Some foods can improve the condition while others can make it worse or interfere with medications.

This book will discuss how diet affects hypothyroidism, which foods to eat and avoid, and examples of a 1-week meal plan. We also look at how the condition affects a person's weight.

While diet cannot cure hypothyroidism, it plays three main roles in managing the condition:

   a. Foods that contain certain nutrients can help maintain proper thyroid function, such as iodine, selenium, and zinc.

   b. Other foods interfere with normal thyroid function, such as those containing goitrogens and soy, so limiting these can improve symptoms.

c. Some foods and supplements can interfere with how well the body absorbs thyroid replacement medicine, so limiting these foods can also help.

Hypothyroidism can lead to weight gain because it can slow down a person's metabolism.

Therefore, a person with hypothyroidism should aim for a healthful diet to prevent weight gain.

Making dietary changes can have an impact on how a person feels and may help improve their quality of life.

The following sections identifies some of the nutrients that can help people with hypothyroidism, and which foods contain them.

Iodine

The body requires iodine to produce thyroid hormones. However, the body cannot make iodine, so a person needs to get iodine from their diet.

Iodine deficiency can also cause an enlarged thyroid gland, known as a goiter. Cheese is rich in iodine, which may help manage hypothyroidism.

Foods rich in iodine include:

- cheese
- milk
- ice cream
- iodized table salt
- saltwater fish

- seaweed
- whole eggs

Iodine deficiency is relatively uncommon in the United States due to the use of iodized table salt, but it is more common in other areas around the world.

However, a person should avoid consuming large amounts of iodine because excess iodine can worsen hypothyroidism and hyperthyroidism.

Selenium

Brazil nuts are rich in selenium.

Selenium is a micronutrient that plays a role in the production of thyroid hormones and has antioxidant activity. The thyroid tissue naturally contains selenium.

Foods rich in selenium include:

- Brazil nuts
- tuna
- shrimp
- beef
- turkey
- chicken
- ham
- eggs
- oatmeal

- whole wheat bread

Zinc

Zinc is another nutrient that has beneficial effects on a person's thyroid hormones.

One small-scale research study showed that zinc supplementation, both alone or in combination with selenium, significantly increased levels of thyroid hormones called T3 and T4.

Foods rich in zinc include:

- oysters
- beef
- crab
- fortified cereal

- chicken
- legumes
- pumpkin seeds
- yogurt

List of foods to avoid and why

Some foods contain nutrients that can interfere with thyroid health. While these foods are not off-limits, people may notice improvements by limiting their consumption.

Goitrogens

Some foods contain goitrogens that can potentially decrease thyroid hormone production.

Foods that contain goitrogens are typically green, cruciferous vegetables, including:

- collards
- brussels sprouts
- Russian kale
- broccoli
- broccoli rabe
- cauliflower
- cabbage

However, these foods also offer plenty of health benefits.

People with hypothyroidism can still enjoy these foods in moderation because scientists believe goitrogens only affect a person's hormones when they consume them in excess.

Also, the cooking process appears to deactivate the goitrogen's effects.

Gluten

Hypothyroidism may have links to an underlying autoimmune disorder, so people may be more at risk of developing other autoimmune conditions, including celiac disease.

Celiac disease causes chronic inflammation and damage to the small intestine due to the ingestion of gluten. Gluten is a protein in wheat and other grains, including barley, oat, and rye.

Treating celiac disease involves following a gluten-free diet. People with autoimmune-related hypothyroidism can try to cut gluten out of their diets to see if their symptoms improve.

Soy

Researchers have found that soy may interfere with how the body produces thyroid hormone.

In one published case study, a woman developed severe hypothyroidism after consuming a health drink containing high amounts of soy for 6 months. Her condition improved after discontinuing the drink and taking thyroid hormone replacement medication.

Foods that contain soy include:

- soy milk
- soy sauce
- edamame
- tofu
- miso
- Processed foods

A person should avoid processed foods, which tend to be calorie-dense and offer little nutritional benefit. These types of foods also promote weight gain.

Examples of processed foods include:

- fast food
- hot dogs

- donuts
- cakes
- cookies

Other diet tips

Certain foods and supplements can make hypothyroid medication less effective.

The following medications and supplements may interfere with the body's absorption of thyroid hormone:

    a. antacids or acid reducers

    b. calcium supplements

    c. iron supplements

    d. high-fiber foods, such as bran flakes, fiber bars, and drinks

  e. foods high in iodine

  f. soy-based foods

People using these medications, supplements, or foods regularly should speak to their doctor regarding the best ways to manage their medication and thyroid hormone levels.

Tips for weight loss with hypothyroidism

People with hypothyroidism may find that they gain weight more easily than people without the condition. This is because hypothyroidism can lower a person's metabolism.

A person with hypothyroidism should focus on a healthful diet rich in fruits, vegetables, and lean proteins. These foods are lower in calories and help keep a person fuller longer, which can help people to maintain a healthful weight.

Regular moderate- to high-intensity aerobic exercise can help increase a person's metabolism to promote weight loss. Doing more activities can also lead to improved energy and sleep.

A person with hypothyroidism can aim for a healthful diet that supports thyroid hormone metabolism and also helps maintain a healthful weight.

Hypothyroidism has links to an underlying autoimmune disorder. It can cause a low metabolism, which leads to easier weight gain. People can treat hypothyroidism with thyroid hormone replacement drugs.

Some foods and nutrients can help or hinder proper thyroid function.

A low thyroid diet ranks top among the major concerns for people with hypothyroidism. Two symptoms of hypothyroidism can have a direct link to your diet. One is unwanted weight gain. The second is that some types of food could trigger a reaction in your thyroid gland. From these two, you can only conclude that a hypothyroid diet is necessary. Your doctor will give you the dos and don'ts for your hypothyroid diet but wouldn't it be nice if it's accompanied by recipes and tips.

Hypothyroidism and Weight Loss Diet

This meal plan helps make life easier (and more delicious) when learning what you should and should not eat with an underactive thyroid.

It's designed to be simple to follow for busy folks with many mouths to feed and realistic, with recipes that beginners can master.

The diet is Gluten-free and loaded with nutrient-dense foods. Naturally rich in selenium, zinc and iodine for thyroid health, and vitamin B12 for more energy.

Ultimately, it is Budget-friendly (except for two worthwhile investments: chia seeds and quinoa).

You can follow the entire plan or simply choose your favourite recipes and include them into your current diet. Many are recipes from qualified Dietitians that I strongly encourage you to follow.

Note that if you are trying to lose a lot of weight, I recommend you read this guide. Also, this is not suitable for those following the Autoimmune Protocol.

Consult with your Personal Doctor or Dietitian first:

While I am a qualified Dietitian, I'm not familiar with your personal medical history, your current medications or additional factors that need to be considered when altering your diet or fitness regime.

Thyroid hormone should be consumed fasting:

At least 1-2 hours before your first food (being conservative). This could mean you skip breakfast altogether, which is fine if it suits you. It just depends on your eating habits and what works best for your lifestyle.

Goitrogens, Soy and Legumes:

Goitrogens and soy seem to be safe in moderate amounts, but you can always leave them out. The same goes for legumes, often left out of Paleo diets (although I don't recommend they be left out). If legumes give you digestive stress, it could be the FODMAPs.

Choose water as your drink:

The meal plan does not include drinks, but keep a bottle of water with you at all times and drink up. Tea is also fine, but anecdotal reports suggest more than 300 mg per day of caffeine (2-3 regular coffees) can aggravate the thyroid.

Flexibility is key:

Of course, this plan cannot meet all your individual needs, so if there is an ingredient you don't eat then replace it or leave it out. Also, it pays off to batch prepare some meals ahead of time so you can simply reheat and go.

Limit or eliminate junk foods and highly processed products:

This plan focuses on whole, unrefined foods as they are fundamental to a healthy diet. Realistically it's very difficult to eliminate all highly processed (often pre-packaged) foods, but just be mindful of cutting down. Likewise, snacks listed are optional depending on your regular eating habits, and there are bonus snack recipe ideas.

The recipes sourced often make 2-4 servings: Consider this when writing your shopping list. You will have leftovers. Feed the family or save the leftovers to have in place of a meal on another day. Recipes toward the end of the week factor in leftovers.

Hypothyroidism diet Preparation Plan for the week

Day 1: Monday

Breakfast: 1 large Banana.

Remember only have breakfast at least 1-2 hours after taking thyroid hormone.

Lunch: Greek Yogurt Tuna Salad. Greek yogurt is high protein and low sugar, while tuna is a rich source of iodine and healthy omega-3 fats.

Dinner: Healthy Chipotle Chicken Sweet Potato Skins. Sweet potato is just one of my all time favourite foods.

Snack: 2-3 Brazil nuts. High in protein, fibre and healthy fats, Brazil nuts are a fantastic source of selenium (for thyroid health). What's more, the addition of nuts to the diet does not increase body weight.

Day 2: Tuesday

Breakfast: Overnight Chocolate Chia Pudding. Chia seeds are a wonderful source of protein, fibre and magnesium. As the name implies, this should be made ahead of time in large batches.

Lunch: Gluten-free sandwich with tinned tuna (or your favourite sandwich topping).

Dinner: Egg Shakshuka + rice to serve. This Tunisian dish is a wonderful source of vegetables and eggs, a source of iodine. Plus rice is naturally gluten-free.

Snack: 1 cup of carrot and cucumber sticks + cottage cheese or hummus (DIY Spicy Peanut Butter Hummus).

Day 3: Wednesday

Breakfast: Gluten-free toast with eggs over-easy.

Lunch: Middle-Eastern Mason Jar Salad. So smart and so simple. Mason jar optional of course, but you need a jar of some type.

Dinner: Shrimp, Zucchini & Pesto Angel Hair Pasta. You should choose gluten-free pasta for this recipe (doesn't need to be angel hair). Shrimp is a good source of iodine.

Snack: 1 banana.

Day 4: Thursday

Breakfast: Green Monster Smoothie. Again, this requires a blender and is another way to make use of your chia seeds, but brush your teeth before work!

Lunch: Pumpkin Soup Like You've Never Tasted Before. I'm a big fan of soups, especially in winter. They tend to be lower-calorie than regular meals, rich in vegetables, and can keep you full for longer.

Dinner: Leftovers.

Snack: 2-3 Brazil nuts.

Day 5: Friday

Breakfast: Choose your favourite.

Lunch: Choose your favourite or leftovers.

Dinner: One Pot Cheesy Taco Skillet. For some reason I like the idea of Mexican on Friday nights, and this creates a fun, communal feel that your family will enjoy.

Snack: 1 cup of carrot and cucumber sticks + cottage cheese or hummus.

Day 6: Saturday

Lunch: Quinoa Salad with Nuts. Quinoa is a versatile grain that is naturally gluten-free and high protein. This recipe has many tasty alternatives depending on what vegetables and nuts you have leftover.

Dinner: Choose your favourite / leftovers / eating out

Snack: Paleo Sweet Potato Fritters

Day 7: Sunday

Breakfast: California Sweet Potato Hash with Feta and Eggs. Because it's Sunday. And sweet potato is good at breakfast too.

Lunch: Choose your favourite / leftovers / eating out

Dinner: Quinoa Crusted Chicken Parmesan + vegetables to serve. Delicious way to serve chicken (you can use regular milk if lactose is no problem for you), and you can make use of any leftover vegetables and cheese.

Snack: 200g (7oz) plain Greek yoghurt + 1 small banana

Hypothyroidism meal plan: 7 days

The best diet for a person with hypothyroidism contains plenty of fruits, vegetables, lean proteins, and a moderate amount of healthful carbohydrates. Salad with grilled shrimp is a recommended lunch on the hypothyroidism meal plan.

Here is an example of a one-week meal plan for a person with hypothyroidism to follow:

Monday

Breakfast: Scrambled eggs with cheddar cheese and whole wheat or gluten-free toast

Lunch: Salad with grilled shrimp

Dinner: Beef stir-fry with vegetables and brown rice.

Tuesday

Breakfast: Oatmeal with berries

Lunch: Grilled chicken salad topped with pumpkin seeds

Dinner: Baked salmon with roasted vegetables

Wednesday

Breakfast: Omelet with mushroom, zucchini, and cheese

Lunch: Bean soup with a whole wheat or gluten-free roll. Recipe here.

Dinner: Beef fajitas with peppers and onions with corn tortillas

Thursday

Breakfast: Plain Greek yogurt with granola and berries

Lunch: Turkey and cheese sandwich on whole wheat or gluten-free bread

Dinner: Roasted chicken with baked beans

Friday

Breakfast: Smoothie with yogurt, banana, and strawberries. Recipe here.

Lunch: Canned tuna with whole wheat or gluten-free crackers

Dinner: Grilled steak with a side salad

Saturday

Breakfast: Fortified cereal with yogurt and fruit

Lunch: Turkey burger on a whole wheat or gluten-free bun

Dinner: Pan-fried crab cakes with brown rice and vegetables.

Sunday

Breakfast: Frittata with vegetables

Lunch: Chicken salad sandwich on a whole wheat or gluten-free bun.

Dinner: Grilled shrimp skewers with bell peppers and pineapple

Hypothyroidism Treatment | Natural Alternatives to Try

1. Iodine

According to observational studies, even a small amount of supplementary iodine can cause a slight, but notable, change in your thyroid gland function. Eating these foods rich in iodine can help prevent iodine deficiency:

- Fish
- Sea vegetables
- Seaweeds
- Eggs
- Berries
- Raw dairy

But, if seafood and dairy are not an option for you, consider taking an all-natural thyroid supplement that contains iodine and other ingredients that target each thyroid symptom. On the other hand, patients with Hashimoto's thyroiditis should not take iodine supplements because getting too much iodine over an extended period can increase the danger of developing an overactive thyroid or other thyroid problems.

The recommended iodine intake is 150-300 μg daily.

2. Selenium

Of all the organs in the body, the thyroid has the highest level of selenium. It is a significant component in the production of the T3 thyroid hormone and can greatly lessen autoimmune effects.

An adequate amount of selenium in our body helps in efficient thyroid hormone synthesis and metabolism. It also decreases anti-thyroid antibody levels and protects the thyroid gland from damage due to radioactive iodine exposures.

The average selenium intake should be 55 μg per day. Salmon, Brazil nuts, beef, sunflower seeds, mushrooms, and onions are some of the foods with high selenium content.

They are also a great addition to your natural hypothyroidism treatment.

3. Vitamin B-Complex

Thiamine and vitamin B12 are essential for hormonal balance and treatment of hypothyroidism.

Vitamin B12 is a vital component for red blood cell production, protein conversion, neurological functions, nerve health, deoxyribonucleic acid (DNA), and fatty acid synthesis. This natural hypothyroidism treatment turns nutrients from food into usable energy for our brain and body.

On the other hand, thiamine can fight the signs and symptoms of autoimmune disease in patients, such as chronic fatigue.

Foods rich in vitamin B-complex include milk, meat, liver, eggs, whole grain cereals, yeast, yogurt, fruits, and green leafy vegetables. One capsule of vitamin B-complex a day is very much required and can be a great treatment for hypothyroidism.

4. Ashwagandha

Adaptogen herbs or supplements like ashwagandha can lower cortisol and balance hormone TSH levels. This herb helps our body respond to stress.

In a clinical trial, supplementing ashwagandha for eight weeks helped patients with hypothyroidism increase their thyroxine hormone levels when compared to using other adaptogen herbs such as Rhodiola, ginseng, licorice root, and holy basil or tulsi, which have comparable benefits.

5. L-Tyrosine

Tyrosine is an amino acid found in our body used by neurotransmitters in our brain and is important for thyroid dysfunction and reduces the risk of thyroid disorders. Supplementing it with L-tyrosine can improve sleep deprivation and fight fatigue and a poor mood by enhancing alertness.

Another reason why it is beneficial in hypothyroidism treatment is it plays a major role in the production of dopamine and melatonin. They are our body's natural "feel-good" hormones.

The recommended dosage of the L-tyrosine supplement is 150 mg/kg per day.

6. Fish Oil

Fish oil capsules are powerful supplements for the brain. Docosahexaenoic acid (DHA) and eicosapentaenoic acid (EPA) omega-3 fatty acids found in fish oil are vital for our brain and thyroid function. They can lower the risk for thyroid disease and symptoms such as depression, anxiety, inflammatory bowel disease, high cholesterol, diabetes, arthritis, a weak immune system, and autoimmune disease.

Fish oil is a powerful brain support nutrient, which is a significant building block for optimal cognitive function. The recommended dosage of this natural hypothyroidism treatment is 1,000 µg daily.

7. Essential Oil

Frankincense, lemongrass, and myrrh essential oils can improve thyroid function and heal symptoms of autoimmune disease. Rubbing these oils directly to the thyroid area along with the reflexology points on the feet and the wrists multiple times a day can offer outstanding relief from pain.

A soothing bath using therapeutic-grade essential oils can also combat fatigue. It can relieve muscle or joint pain, improve mood, and reduce anxiety and irritability as well.

8. Acupuncture

This traditional Chinese medicine is popular for alleviating pain and improving symptoms of different health conditions like hypothyroidism.

Acupuncture uses needles to prick the skin to target various pressure points in the body.

It helps regulate the flow of energy and correct variances in the body, such as hormonal imbalance. One study revealed that people who have thyroid dysfunction experienced improvements in their thyroid hormone markers when they applied acupuncture therapy regularly.

It also allows you to relax and aids in relieving anxiety and muscle tension, which are both hypothyroidism symptoms. Ask your doctor how you can incorporate acupuncture in your hypothyroidism treatment.

9. Probiotics

Your gut is a large reservoir of thyroid hormones where the good bacteria in there help convert T3 to T4, which is often deficient in hypothyroidism. Try taking probiotics with Lactobacillus bacteria for your thyroid health.

How to Lower Your Risk of Hypothyroidism

Hypothyroidism and other types of thyroid disease are generally not preventable as they are, most of the time, autoimmune. But in cases not relating to genetic makeup, there are risk factors that can predispose one to hypothyroidism.

They are preventable though. The following are best practices to help keep a healthy thyroid:

1. Manage Stress

Chronic stress can trigger thyroid dysfunction as excess cortisol from it prevents your thyroid from making more hormones.

On top of that, stress can worsen the condition's symptoms if you already have an underactive thyroid. This is why it's important to know how to manage stress to prevent thyroid problems.

Practice self-care to control stress. You can try these activities:

- Book reading
- Walking outside
- Taking a bath with essential oils
- Having a massage
- Performing meditation

It's crucial to make time to relax each day. If it's difficult for you to do so, start with two or three times a week and then increase the number of days as you go until you can finally make it to every day.

2. Minimize Sugar Consumption

Too much sugar may trigger yeast overgrowth which has been linked to Hashimoto's disease, the most common cause of hypothyroidism.

Aside from that, your thyroid is also responsible for regulating the metabolism of carbs. If there is low hormone production or central hypothyroidism, your body will have a difficult time balancing your blood sugar levels, leading to metabolic issues, weight gain, or fatigue.

3. Avoid Gluten in Your Hypothyroidism Diet

Go for gluten-free loaves of bread to keep your thyroid healthy.

Gluten is a type of protein present in grains like rye, barley, and wheat. It may cause damage to your gut lining, interrupting thyroid hormone activities and causing inflammation that can reach your thyroid.

The manufacturing of gluten includes bromide, which takes over iodine. You can ask your doctor how you can go gluten-free in your hypothyroidism diet plan to keep your thyroid healthy.

4. Watch Out for Perchlorates

Perchlorates are a type of odorless and colorless salt used in making fireworks and explosives. They can contaminate water systems. High levels of this chemical can lower your TSH levels as it blocks your thyroid from absorbing iodine. Consider having your water tested for perchlorates.

5. Quit Smoking

Smoking is never good for your health as it leaves various types of toxins in your body. The chemical thiocyanate in cigarettes can interfere with your thyroid's absorption of iodine, blocking the production of thyroid hormones.

Quitting smoking may be difficult, so you might need your doctor's involvement to help you with this. If you're a non-smoker, it's best to not try smoking at all.

6. Perform a Thyroid Neck Check

A thyroid neck check is a test you can do at home to see if there are bumps in your thyroid area that may be a symptom of the condition.

To do the test, follow these steps:

Use a mirror and hold it in your hand, reflecting the lower front area of your neck where your thyroid is.

Tip your head back while you take a look at your neck in the mirror.

Drink water and watch your neck closely as you swallow.

Check if you see bulges in the area of your neck closer to your collarbone upon swallowing the water.

If you see something, consult your doctor right away as it may indicate inflammation in your thyroid.

7. See Your Physician Regularly

On top of doing a thyroid neck check, it's also essential to visit your doctor for a thyroid checkup. This is highly recommended if you think you are experiencing symptoms of the condition or you have a family history of hypothyroidism or any related thyroid disease.

If several members of the family have thyroid issues, your doctor will likely want to perform thyroid tests to monitor your thyroid hormones yearly.

Hypothyroidism is a condition that should not be taken lightly because it can get serious. Conventional medicines can cure the disorder, but there's a possibility that it can affect other organs and their functions.

This can lead to a more critical condition. Using natural hypothyroidism treatment can be just as effective as modern medicines but doesn't have harmful side effects.

Some pharmaceutical drugs can have adverse reactions in patients who take them. Herbal or natural medicines utilize our body's natural healing process, and they are more cost-effective compared to modern medicines.

Everyone is prone to developing thyroid problems due to age, diet, and stress. Thyroid conditions may also be healed with simple remedies. One of these great remedies includes this amazing gut-healing smoothie may visibly improve your thyroid health. A low thyroid diet or even a treatment plan for hyperthyroidism may be better optimized with this wonder smoothie.

Fill your gut with goodness with this probiotic rich breakfast smoothie. A gut brimming with probiotics can boost your entire system. Make this smoothie and enjoy its benefits.

Banana Turmeric Peanut Butter

Ingredients

- 1 tbsp peanut butter
- 1 tbsp ground turmeric
- A dash black pepper

- 3 tbsp ginger finely chopped
- A small banana
- ¼ cup blueberries
- 1 tsp chia seeds
- t tsp hemp powder
- ¼ cup greek yogurt
- ¼ cup oats
- 1 cup unsweetened almond milk

Preparation

1. Combine ingredients and spin in a blender until blended smooth.
2. Add more liquid to make it creamier, or ice to make it chunkier.

Turmeric Tea Recipe For A Healthy Thyroid

Turmeric has been historically known for its many health benefits, and this simple turmeric tea recipe may help you optimize your thyroid treatment plan. Turmeric health benefits include improved oxygen intake and low cholesterol levels which makes this recipe extremely good for your thyroid.

Turmeric Tea Recipe for Your Thyroid

Ingredients

- Turmeric powder (1-2 tbsp)
- Black pepper powder (1 tsp)

- Boiling water (1 cup)
- Virgin coconut oil (1 tsp)
- Sliced ginger
- Cinnamon

Step 1: Prepare Turmeric Powder

Prepare your turmeric powder, about half a teaspoon. Put this in a small cup.

The long list of turmeric health benefits includes anti-inflammation, low cholesterol levels, weight loss, and detox. This powder also has thyroid-specific benefits such as increased thyroid levels and may prevent thyroid cancer.

Step 2: Add Black Pepper Powder

This additional ingredient may help enhance the benefits of the turmeric. Black pepper has been known to increase the bioavailability of the turmeric powder by allowing your body to make the most of the turmeric's curcumin content.

Step 3: Fill the Cup with Boiling Water

Once the turmeric and black pepper are in a small cup, fill the cup with boiling water. The boiling water will dissolve the pepper and turmeric. Make sure to stir the tea to let the ingredients mix together in the cup.

Step 4: Add in Virgin Coconut Oil

Add a teaspoon of virgin coconut oil. This oil may also help your body absorb the curcumin with ease because turmeric has been known to be better absorbed when taken with fat soluble. Virgin coconut oil may also help you maintain a healthy thyroid gland because of its fatty acids.

Step 5: Try Mixing in Ginger

To add some extra taste and thyroid health benefits to this turmeric tea recipe, put in a few slices of ginger. Ginger is especially great for inflammation and improving thyroid function. It may also help your thyroid regulate your metabolism.

Step 6: Add Cinnamon for Taste

Sprinkle some cinnamon powder on top of your turmeric tea. The cinnamon will add some taste to the tea and help with your hypothyroidism. Just like the ginger, it also has anti-inflammatory properties. It may also help regulate your body's sugar levels to prevent diabetes.

Step 7: Drink this Tea Regularly

You may try this turmeric tea recipe twice a day, once in the morning and before you go to sleep.

Try it for two weeks then take a two-day break before continuing this routine.

Strawberry-Almond-Coconut Smoothie

Ingredients:

- 2 tablespoons unsalted almond butter
- 3/4 cup unsweetened coconut milk
- 1/2 cup unsweetened almond milk
- 1/2 cup frozen organic strawberries
- 2 teaspoons chia seeds
- 1 or 2 large ice cubes

Preparation:

1. Blend all ingredients at high speed until it reaches your desired texture.
2. Add a little filtered water if it's too thick then blend again.

Cocoa Bliss Smoothie

Ingredients

- 1 cup almond or cashew milk
- 1 tablespoon raw cacao powder
- 1/2 cup full fat coconut milk
- 1 tablespoon coconut butter
- 1 teaspoon no alcohol pure vanilla

Preparation:

1. Combine all ingredients in a blender.
2. Blend until creamy and smooth.

If you're not a big fan of smoothies, you might want to try juices. These are easier to consume along with your meals given that they aren't as thick as smoothies. Here is an easy recipe for a juice you could have at home:

Watercress Green Juice

Ingredients:

- 2 cups of watercress leaves and stems
- 2 red or green apples

- a squeeze of lemon juice

Preparation:

- Combine all ingredients in a juicer.
- Serve with ice.

Note: Drink in moderation. Watercress is highly detoxifying.

Rosemary Roasted Potatoes and Tomatoes

Just because salads are healthy, doesn't mean they have to be ho hum. Try this lively combination of roasted new potatoes, fresh rosemary, tomatoes, kalamata olives, and Parmesan cheese.

SERVINGS: 8 | **TOTAL TIME**: 35 min

Ingredients

- 1 pound potatoes, new (tiny) scrubbed and quartered
- 2 tablespoons oil, olive
- 1 teaspoon rosemary, snipped
- ¼ teaspoon salt
- ¼ teaspoon pepper, black, ground
- 4 tomatoes, plum, quartered lengthwise
- ½ cup olives, Kalamata, pitted, halved
- 3 cloves garlic, minced
- ¼ cup cheese, Parmesan grated

Instructions

1. Preheat oven to 450°F. Lightly grease a 15x10x1-inch baking pan; place potatoes in pan.
2. In a small bowl, combine oil, rosemary, salt, and pepper; drizzle over potatoes, tossing to coat.
3. Bake for 20 minutes, stirring once. Add tomatoes, olives, and garlic, tossing to combine. Bake for 5 to 10 minutes more or until potatoes are tender and brown on the edges and tomatoes are soft.

4. Transfer to a serving dish. Sprinkle with Parmesan cheese.

Nutrition Details (per serving)

Calories 103, Fat 5g, Cholesterol 2mg, Sodium 208mg, Saturated Fat 1g, Protein 3g, Fiber 2g, Carbohydrates 11g

Baked Risotto Primavera

This updated spring classic calls for nutty-tasting short-grain brown rice instead of the traditional white Arborio. Because the cooking time is longer with whole-grain rice, this risotto is cooked in the oven rather than on the stovetop, eliminating the need for almost constant stirring.

SERVINGS: 6 | **TOTAL TIME**: 1 hr 25 min

Ingredients

- 1 tablespoon oil, olive, extra-virgin
- 2 medium onions chopped, (about 1 ½ cups)
- 1 cup rice, brown medium- or short-grain
- 3 cloves garlic minced
- ½ cup wine, dry white
- 29 ounces broth, chicken, less sodium or 3 ½ cups vegetable broth
- 8 ounces asparagus ends trimmed, cut into 1-inch pieces
- 1 cup peas, sugar snap or snow peas, trimmed, cut into 1-inch pieces

- 1 cup peppers, red, bell diced, (about 1 medium)
- 1 ½ cups cheese, Parmesan freshly grated
- ¼ cup parsley, fresh chopped
- ¼ cup chives, fresh chopped
- 2 teaspoon lemon zest (1 - 2 teaspoons as desired)
- pepper, black ground to taste

Instructions

1. Preheat oven to 425 degrees F.
2. Heat oil in a Dutch oven or ovenproof high sided skillet over medium heat. Add onions

and cook, stirring occasionally, until softened, 3 to 5 minutes.

3. Stir in rice and garlic; cook, stirring, 1 to 2 minutes. Stir in wine and simmer until it has mostly evaporated. Add broth and bring to a boil. Cover the pan and transfer to the oven.
4. Bake until the rice is just tender, 50 minutes to 1 hour.
5. Shortly before the risotto is done, steam asparagus, peas, and bell pepper until crisp-tender, about 4 minutes.
6. Fold the steamed vegetables, Parmesan, parsley, chives, lemon zest, and pepper into the risotto. Serve immediately.

Nutrition Details (per serving)

Calories 267, Fat 8g, Cholesterol 11mg, Sodium 607mg, Saturated Fat 3g, Protein 12g, Fiber 4g, Carbohydrates 35g

Southwestern Steak and Peppers

This juicy spice-crusted steak gets finished with a dynamite sauce made with an unusual ingredient — coffee, which adds depth and richness to the dish. Slice the steak very thinly across the grain to ensure the most tender results.

SERVINGS: 4 | **TOTAL TIME**: 30 min

Ingredients

- ½ tablespoon cumin, ground
- ½ teaspoon coriander, ground
- ½ teaspoon chili powder
- ¼ teaspoon salt
- ¾ teaspoon pepper, black, coarsely ground
- 1 pound beef, boneless top sirloin steak trimmed of fat
- 3 cloves garlic, peeled, 1 halved and 2 minced
- 3 teaspoons oil, canola divided (or olive oil)
- 2 medium peppers, red, bell thinly sliced

- 1 medium onion, white halved lengthwise and thinly sliced
- 1 teaspoon sugar, brown
- 1/2 cups coffee, brewed or prepared instant coffee
- 1/4 cup vinegar, balsamic
- 4 cups watercress

Instructions

1. Mix cumin, coriander, chili powder, salt, and 3/4 teaspoon pepper in a small bowl. Rub steak with the cut garlic. Rub the spice mix all over the steak.

2. Heat 2 teaspoons oil in a large heavy skillet, preferably cast iron, over medium-high heat. Add the steak and cook to desired doneness, 4 to 6 minutes per side for medium-rare. Transfer to a cutting board and let rest.

3. Add remaining 1 teaspoon oil to the skillet. Add bell peppers and onion; cook, stirring often, until softened, about 4 minutes.

4. Add minced garlic and brown sugar; cook, stirring often, for 1 minute. Add coffee, vinegar, and any accumulated meat juices; cook for 3 minutes to intensify flavor. Season with pepper.

5. To serve, mound 1 cup watercress on each plate. Top with the sautéed peppers and

onion. Slice the steak thinly across the grain and arrange on the vegetables.

6. Pour the sauce from the pan over the steak. Serve immediately.

Nutrition Details (per serving)

Calories 226, Fat 12g, Cholesterol 60mg, Sodium 216mg, Saturated Fat 3g, Protein 26g, Fiber 3g, Carbohydrates 12g

Sizzled Citrus Shrimp

This quick Spanish-inspired sauté is a lesson in simplicity. All shrimp really needs to dazzle is lots of garlic and a splash of lemon. Serve as a main dish or as a tapa (appetizer).

SERVINGS: 4 | **TOTAL TIME**: 30 min

Ingredients

- 3 tablespoons lemon juice
- 3 tablespoons wine, dry white
- 2 teaspoons oil, olive, extra-virgin
- 3 cloves garlic minced
- 1 pound shrimp, peeled and deveined medium (30-40 per pound)
- 1 teaspoon oil, olive, extra-virgin
- 1 whole bay leaf

- 1/4 teaspoon pepper, red, crushed or 1 dried red chile, halved
- 1/4 teaspoon salt or to taste
- 2 tablespoons parsley, fresh chopped

Instructions

1. Combine lemon juice, wine, 2 teaspoons oil, and garlic in a medium bowl. Add shrimp and toss to coat. Cover and marinate in the refrigerator for 15 minutes, tossing occasionally. Drain well, reserving marinade.
2. Heat 1 teaspoon oil in a large nonstick skillet over medium-high heat. Add shrimp and cook, turning once, until barely pink, about 30 seconds per side; transfer to a plate.

3. Add bay leaf, crushed red pepper, and the reserved marinade to the pan; simmer for 4 minutes. Return the shrimp and any accumulated juices to the pan; heat through.
4. Season with salt, sprinkle with parsley, and serve immediately.

Nutrition Details (per serving)

Calories 171, Fat 6g, Cholesterol 172mg, Sodium 315mg, Saturated Fat 1g, Protein 23g, Fiber 1g, Carbohydrates 4g

Ginger-Chicken Noodle Soup

SERVINGS: 5 | **TOTAL TIME**: 48 min

Ingredients

- 1 pound chicken, thighs skinless, boneless, cut into 1-inch pieces
- 1 tablespoon oil, cooking
- 2 medium carrots cut into thin bite-size sticks
- 3 cans broth, chicken, less sodium 14 ounces each
- 1 cup water
- 2 tablespoons vinegar, rice
- 1 tablespoon soy sauce, less sodium

- 2 ½ teaspoons ginger, fresh
- ¼ teaspoon pepper, black, ground
- 2 ounces rice noodles, dried
- 6 ounces pea pods, frozen, thawed, and halved diagonally

Instructions

1. In a Dutch oven, cook chicken, half at a time, in hot oil just until browned. Drain fat. Return all chicken to Dutch oven. Add carrots, broth, water, vinegar, soy sauce, ginger, and pepper. Bring to boiling; reduce heat and simmer, covered, 20 minutes.

2. Return to boil. Add noodles. Simmer, uncovered, 8 to 10 minutes or until noodles

are tender, adding pea pods the last 1 to 2 minutes. If desired serve with additional soy sauce.

Nutrition Details (per serving)

Calories 221, Fat 6g, Cholesterol 72mg, Sodium 805mg, Saturated Fat 1g, Protein 23g, Fiber 2g, Carbohydrates 16g

Green Beans With Bacon and Hazelnuts

The toasted smoky flavors in this fast sauté make it a warm addition to any winter meal.

SERVINGS: 4 | TOTAL TIME: 20 min

Ingredients

- 1 teaspoon oil, canola
- 1 large shallot minced
- 1 pound beans, green trimmed
- 1/2 cup water
- 2 slices bacon cooked and crumbled
- 2 tablespoons nuts, hazelnuts toasted, chopped
- 1/4 teaspoon salt

Instructions

1. Heat oil in a large skillet over medium-high heat. Add shallot and cook, stirring, until starting to brown, 30 seconds to 1 minute.

2. Add green beans and cook, stirring often, until seared in spots, 2 to 3 minutes.

3. Add water; cover, reduce heat to medium and cook, stirring occasionally, about 3 minutes for tender-crisp or 6 minutes for tender. Remove from heat and stir in bacon, hazelnuts, and salt.

Nutrition Details (per serving)

Calories 100, Fat 5g, Cholesterol 3mg, Sodium 226mg, Saturated Fat 1g, Protein 5g, Fiber 4g, Carbohydrates 12g

Smoky Stuffed Peppers

Turkey sausage and smoked cheese give a flavorful boost to this versatile, somewhat retro dinner. We've speeded it up by microwave-blanching the peppers and using instant brown rice. If possible, choose peppers that will stand upright.

SERVINGS: 6 | **TOTAL TIME**: 45 min

Ingredients

- 6 large peppers, bell, any color tops cut off, seeded
- 12 ounces sausage, Italian turkey, hot links, removed from casings

- 1 ½ cups broth, chicken, less sodium
- 4 medium tomatoes, plum chopped
- 2 cups rice, brown, instant
- 1 cup basil, fresh chopped
- 1 cup cheese, smoked mozzarella (or smoked cheddar or Gouda), finely shredded, divided

Instructions

1. Position rack in upper third of oven; preheat broiler.
2. Place peppers cut-side down in a large microwave-safe dish. Fill the dish with 1/2 inch of water, cover and microwave on High until the peppers are just softened, 7 to 10

minutes. Drain the water and transfer the peppers to a roasting pan.

3. Meanwhile, cook sausage in a large nonstick skillet over medium-high heat, breaking it up into small pieces with a wooden spoon, until cooked through, about 5 minutes.

4. Stir in broth, tomatoes, and rice; increase heat to high and bring to a simmer. Cover, reduce heat to medium-low and simmer until the rice is softened but still moist, 5 minutes. Remove from the heat and let stand, covered, until the rice absorbs the remaining liquid, about 5 minutes.

5. Stir basil and half the cheese into the rice mixture. Divide the filling among the

peppers, then top with the remaining cheese. Broil until the cheese is melted, 2 to 3 minutes.

Nutrition Details (per serving)

Calories 294, Fat 11g, Cholesterol 45mg, Sodium 533mg, Saturated Fat 5g, Protein 19g, Fiber 5g, Carbohydrates 32g

Printed in Great Britain
by Amazon